Plantar Fasciitis: The Best Plantar Fasciitis Survival Guide With Special Tips On How to Manage Heel Spur and Get Plantar Fasciitis Cure Today!

By Brian Jeff

~~~

Copyright © 2016 by Brian Jeff

This ebook is licensed for your personal enjoyment only. This ebook may not be re-sold or given away to other people. If you would like to share this book with another person, please purchase an additional copy for each recipient. If you're reading this book and did not purchase it, or it was not purchased for your use only, then please return it and purchase your own copy. Thank you for respecting the hard work of this author.

Disclaimer

The Publisher has strived to be as accurate and complete as possible in the creation of this report, notwithstanding the fact that the publisher does not warrant or represent at any time that the contents within are accurate due to the rapidly changing nature of the Internet.

While all attempts have been made to verify information provided in this publication, the Publisher assumes no responsibility for errors, omissions, or contrary interpretation of the subject matter herein. Any perceived slights of specific persons, peoples, or organizations are unintentional.

In practical advice books, like anything else in life, there are no guarantees of income made. Readers are cautioned to rely on their own judgment about their individual circumstances to act accordingly.

This book is not intended for use as a source of legal, business, accounting or financial advice. All readers are advised to seek services of competent professionals in legal, business, accounting and financial fields.

Table Of Contents

Overview: Understanding Plantar Fasciitis

Symptoms and Causes of Plantar Fasciitis

Soothing Heal Pain With Plantar Fasciitis Exercise

Heel Spur Symptoms

Best Plantar Fasciitis Treatment

Conclusion

Overview: Understanding Plantar Fasciitis

Without doubt if you know what I am talking about here you will agree with me that Plantar fasciitis is an unpleasant problem that you will not want even your enemy to go through… they are induced pain that manifest under the heel.

As a matter of fact, this condition is commonly known to be induced by overwhelming or overstretching the plantar fascia, also known as the arch tendon of your foot.

Well, besides the above, which are the main triggers of plantar fasciitis … it is known to be triggered by a variety of other things such as the following:

Taking part in a lot of exercise, for instance, including too many kilometers to your strolling or activities, using damaged shoes, and over pronation

Yes, over pronation occurs when standing for a long time…I mean pronation occurs as the foot rolls inside and the arch of the foot crushes, hence the term often used to refer to somebody who over pronates is one who have 'flat feet'.

Now, you need to know that pronation is a normal part of the gait cycle which helps to make available shock absorption at the foot.

So, rolling your foot excessively inward while strolling or walking; and being on your feet all day long could give rise to the condition!

Symptoms of plantar fasciitis

Yes, as for the symptoms… you might struggle with quick discomfort in your foot for starters, especially the heel, where plantar fascia tendon starts its quest to the toes.

The pain is normally even more extreme after long periods of lack of exercise or in the early morning.

As a matter of fact, sufferers may typically experience discomfort at the start of activity, which minimizes or is gotten rid of after conditioning.

Well, the pain can easily also take place after extended standing and then could be accompanied by some rigidity. Anyway, in more severe situations, the pain might worsen at nights.

Plantar fasciitis treatment

To start with, the good news concerning the condition… is that it usually responds to treatment well, but I must add that this is the case if the treatment is started quite early after the beginning of the discomfort.

However, it typically will take 6-8 weeks to overcome it, even though, for most of that time you feel like you will never overcome it.

In any case where you do not get managed well, the disorder could possibly worsen and then you might start experiencing morning discomfort for up to a minimum of a year.

As such, you may not be able to do several of your treasured activities.

Treatment could consist of:
Stretching workouts to improve the size of plantar fascia and also heel wire,

Ice massage under the foot to alleviate heel discomfort,

Using shoes that are flat with soft heels,

Acupuncture,

Physiotherapy by electrical stimulation,

Touching the bottom of injured foot, Now, briefly shift to the other form of exercises like cycling and swimming instead of sports that entail leaping and working.

Equally, you may possibly need to put on a night splint for 6-8 weeks. This assists to maintain your foot in a slightly flexed or neutral position as you rest. It aids to sustain the normal stretch of the heel wire and then plantar fascia.

Besides, there are a number of plantar fasciitis stretches you can easily attempt, such as rolling an icy water bottle or golf ball under the foot in order to soothe the discomfort.

Nonetheless, the doctor might additionally prescribe orthotics to deliver you some feet extra support.

Another alternative is cortisone whacks. However, these can be remarkably uncomfortable and besides that, it will only assist regarding only about fifty percent of the situations. But, in rare situations, surgery could be needed.

Avoidance of plantar fasciitis

Now, besides keeping entirely off your feet, there are a few steps you ought to take in order to minimize your risk of establishing this disorder:

Yes, do not suddenly increase your training tons. Rather, do it steadily. Constantly wear shoes that could support your arch while working out. Make sure you have excellent adaptability around your ankle.

Take note and take good care of your shoes and boots especially when you are not exercising as it is very important!

Only wear comfortable shoes for plantar fasciitis to adequately sustain your arcs.

Moreover, you must ensure you do not go about in thin shoes or barefooted as both could postpone your recuperation.

Symptoms and Causes of Plantar Fasciitis

Yes, with all research results, it has been shown that the most common cause of heel pain is plantar fasciitis, which is also called heel spur syndrome.

Besides, we also know that heel pain also encompasses numerous other ailments of the foot, including nerve irritation, arthritis, tendonitis, stress fracture, and in rare cases, cysts.

But, because there are so many reasons for heel pain, it is always best to get the foot looked at by a medical professional to ascertain the main issue.

In that case, a podiatrist, orthopedic or foot and ankle surgeon is your best bet for a proper diagnosis, as they specialize in problems involving the foot.

Well, the truth is that some heel pain may get better on its own, but in some case, they may worsen off, if people ignore the pain and continue to perform activities that injured it in the first place.

Now, if this happens to anyone, just beware… the heel pain may continue to get worse, and if care is not taken, it can become a chronic condition that will deteriorate over time!

Even so, at these stages, surgery is hardly ever necessary for the scenarios....

However, you must understand though, heel pain effects are insignificant at the starting point, with essentially no torment experienced by you.

Nonetheless, getting an x-ray will clearly demonstrate the true degree of the condition.

Yes, with such procedure, you may recognize a bone-like development in your heel, and that can irritate muscle tissue and ligaments in the event that it keeps on growing to be bigger or greater.

Therefore, recognizing the real presence of a goad right on time, I mean at the early stages makes it conceivable to abstain from feeling ache in situations where your plantar belt or some other ligament encounters aggravation.

Well, be that as it may, it's not in any manner exceptional for both specialists and patients to miss this key window on the grounds that it's simpler to diagnose a goad that as of now causes some volume of uneasiness.

Now, to start the heel torment treatment once you have gotten a legitimate judgment about the issue through proper diagnosis, it will be discerning to think of minimizing the harm the calcium development causes first.

By that I mean your essential objective at this stage will be to reduce the swelling and unwind your tendons and muscles to take into account the recuperation procedure to begin.

Yes, that process could start with an ice pack treatment which is reputed to give transitory alleviation, while at it, letting the swelling on your feet begin to go down.

Well, besides that, distinctive regular home cures including natively constructed blends additionally help bring down the swelling of your own ligaments.

Moreover, joining smashed flaxseed with a bit of water produces the glue that you'll be able to spread on your feet.

At this junction, let me say, there are many treatments for heel pain.

However, most specialists or doctors should be able to customize a treatment plan depending on individual factors including lifestyle, foot types and any other associated illnesses.

By that I mean that treatment should not only concentrate on the heel but also on the person as a whole.

The truth is that at this stage, so many factors both physical and psychological may be important to consider.

In addition, weight control, systemic medical conditions and injuries should be evaluated.

Evaluations consist of a thorough history and physical examination, x-rays, diagnostic ultrasound and MRI if necessary. Referrals to other specialists may be needed if there are associated medical conditions.

After all that, the real treatment may include anti-inflammatory pills, ice, cortisone injections, custom orthotic arch supports, padding, strapping, night splints, removable casts, and stretching.

Besides, it also include, physical therapy, shockwave, homeopathic and natural medicine, change in activities, weight-loss programs, wearing different shoes, and a general change in life style.

Soothing Heal Pain With Plantar Fasciitis Exercise.

There is no doubt that being struck by a pain that is called a plantar fasciitis might be one of those painful experiences in life you may often have to go through.

But the truth is when I was struck by this condition some time ago I know how painful it can be, yes, it was very painful but I did treat it with plantar fasciitis exercises.

Now, I need to be specific, if it is the case that you feel severe pain around your heel in the morning, you might be having a plantar fasciitis.

As a matter of fact, plantar fasciitis is caused when the plantar fascia (the link between your heel bone and your toes) is strained.

And indeed, it is most common for overweight people or people who trek a lot. Yes, the condition does not usually start at once; in fact, it starts gradually unnoticed with a mild pain till it becomes big!

Now, let's face it, if you do not treat a plantar fasciitis, it can become so big that some parts of your body (like knee, foot and back) will be affected and as a result of that fact, it can without doubt alter the way you walk.

It is, however, easy to get yourself treated from this pain easily without going to any physician.

Well, I mean you only need to perform some simple plantar fasciitis exercises and you will get your relief!

Yes, one of the ways you can get rid of this pain is by stretching the plantar fascia. Okay, to stretch it, you will need to pull up on the affected leg for about 30 seconds by stretching five times or three times a day.

What that will do for you is that it will help relieve the pain, although it takes a lot of determination to be able to stretch at the recommended rate.

However, this is one of the treatments that are known to reduce its chances of reoccurring.

Well, in another plantar fasciitis exercises, you can bend your knee with your other knee straight and the heel on the ground while you lean against a wall. As you lean, your foot arch will get stretched.

Now, if you will do this exercise, always do it for 10 seconds with an interval for rest. However, you can do this repeatedly for 20 times with respect to the affected heel.

Another exercise to do is where you can also spread your feet apart with your feet facing each other while you lean forward on a countertop.

Squat down, then flex your knees before you place your feet down for as long as you can. You can do this also for 20 times with an interval after the end of each.

Moreover, another way you can also treat this is with your hand… yes, use your hand to pull your toes back towards your shin while the affected leg is crossed over the other leg.

Yes, without doubt, this action will stretch your plantar fascia, thereafter, you can then check by placing the thumb of your healthy leg on the plantar fascia which is very firm and then rub it gently for about ten times.

Now, I need to warn… though, you need to always stretch fascia, but without doubt, this it is very important, however, what is equally important is that you do not over stretch the affected part.

As a matter of fact, it can be stretched early in the morning or late in the night.

However, if after some months of performing the plantar fasciitis exercise committedly and nothing happens, you may need to see a doctor.

Yes, he/she will make some prescription but I dare say that these plantar fasciitis exercises have a high rate of being successful.

Heel Spur Symptoms

Simply put, the hardened outgrowth on the heel bone is well-known as a heel spur. As a matter of fact, it results to intense heel pain that can make it hard for you to perform your daily operations.

To put it mildly, heel spurs are a very common foot problem in countless people.

Auspiciously, for many people though, there's a reasonable and an efficient heel spur treatment solution for this agonizing foot condition.

Yes, the bone outgrowth tends to lay pressure on the ligament connected to the heel bone, which as a result causes its inflammation!

Well, to be frank with you, the inflammation is the root cause of the heel pain you feel. But, if a heel spur is left unattended, it can tear this ligament and cause more damage!

Now, before you continue, I want you to answer the following questions: Do you suffer from unbearable pain in your heel?

Do you wake up every day with sore feet? Are you not sure that your pain is a symptom of a heel spur?

If your answer to these questions is confirmatory or positive, then go ahead read this!

Yes, it's time to dig deeper… let's take a look at information on how to realize or should I say, identify the heel spur symptoms, in fact, in medical terms, it is referred to as calcaneal spur.

Without doubt, extreme pain in heels can be a very agonizing experience and the reason is not farfetched.

Yes, your feet bear the weight of your body and if your feet pain you badly, you will definitely find it hard to do activities like standing for a long time, walking, lifting heavy objects, climbing a stair or you will be immobilized!

Well, the bad news is that there are numerous medical conditions, such as stressed fracture, nerve damage, tarsal tunnel syndrome, plantar fasciitis, heel spur, arthritis etc. that can result in extreme pain in the heels.

And most of these conditions are interconnected and, hence, it becomes hard to diagnose the real problem.

As a matter of fact, most times, the friction leads to irritation or swelling that usually leaves one with no option than to seek for relief!

Well, the truth is that, heel spur is a common medical condition rampant in people who are in their middle age.

In fact, it is a knob of bone that is formed on the heels. And, like any of the above stated medical conditions, it is also characterized by severe pain in the heel.

Besides, it is the most common heel spur symptom highly reported by the patients.

According to a survey, the majority of the people suffering from heel spur reported having excruciating pain in their heels while taking the first few steps in the morning. Yes, the pain tends to lessen as you walk more and finally it recedes to a dull ache.

So, as you can see, heel spur can't be always painful. In fact, the pain is typically relieved during rest, but the condition is worse after getting up once more.

The pain can develop to be so severe that it becomes hard to carry on your daily operations!

But you need to realize whether …
the pain in the heel is the sign of heel spur or not. This is very important.

In heel spur, the pain is accompanied by bruises and redness. Well, in other cases, patients have reported calluses and corns as signs of a heel spur, along with the pain in the heels.

As a matter of fact, the agony caused by heel spur is like something piercing being stabbed into your heel.

Though, the pain lessens with continuous walking, however, if you take a break or stop in between and sit down, the next time you stand to walk again the pain soars higher.

Now, without doubt, I want you to know that the most important aspect in heel spur treatment is rest, in fact, medics usually advise patients to take enough rest.

Well, fortunately, a heel spur can be treated after diagnoses very easily.

Though at first, it is essential for you to understand the symptom and consult your doctor.

That's simply to say, do not adhere to any treatment formula without the knowledge of your physician or doctor.

Best Plantar Fasciitis Treatment

Most of us who have once experienced plantar fasciitis know clearly how devastating and frustrating the situation can be.

From my experience, every morning completely resembled being forced to walk or make a move on broken glass and you rapidly become dissatisfied and grumpy.

The lifetime occurrence for plantar fasciitis may be as high as 10% which means that quite a large percentage of us will at some point in life be affected by plantar fasciitis.

But typically, a foot pain ailment referred to as plantar fasciitis, develops due to small tears in the area of the feet where back heel connects to the bone.

This may arise as a result of jogging and inappropriate walking strategies.

Well, besides that, an excess of body weight could possibly cause these minute tears to form or grow in size resulting to ever more agony for the individual so affected.

Now, get a fast relief and be secured from this condition, among the top precautionary cures is to put on the proper shoes for plantar fasciitis treatment.

Yes, from my experience I realized using cheaply manufactured sneakers or poorly fitting ones lead to heel pain!

So, when you wear shoes, you want to make sure you choose and pick footwear that actually possess some brilliant padding; as a matter of fact, things like flip flops lead me to plantar fasciitis after using them too much.

Therefore, the best footwear for getting rid of the condition should have no or minimum heel (for ladies, get shoe heels less than two inches long), in fact, a highly shock absorbing sole, and cushioned arch foot support will be perfect.

Unfortunately, the majority of the shoes on the market don't have proper arch support for the heel; without doubt, shoes that don't have an excellent heel and mid-foot foot support may result in plantar fasciitis.

So, I can tell you from my experience that, if you put on the best shoes for plantar fasciitis, you stand a considerably reduced chance of getting heel pain.

Yes, as these shoes are known to have much better heel support for both the heel bone and arch of the foot which may help with the condition.

It is advisable to make connecting your shoe correctly extremely important...

by regularly wearing shoes that do not fit, you will cause plantar fasciitis.

And if you opt to purchase plantar fasciitis shoes, be sure you test them out late in the afternoon, as feet might be bigger in the afternoon than at the beginning of the day.

Furthermore, men and women will have one foot a bit larger than the other.

So, when scouting for shoes, target the padding and support for the bottom of the feet, the back heel, and the front side of the feet.

You ought to ensure that your pair of brand new sneakers is comfortable; the truth is that, you don't need an excessive force on any one single section of your feet.

Besides that, it's also important that you select a pair of shoes which have a larger toe region to minimize any potential problems with hallux valgus.

Anyway, timely diagnosing along with a mapped out treatment plan are very important for curing plantar fasciitis.

The truth is that, if you don't discover plantar fasciitis in their initial phases or stages if you like, it could take about a year or more to get it treated when discovered late!

Well, having said that, curing plantar fasciitis usually does not require an operation, particularly when preventative measures are pursued like wearing the best shoes for plantar fasciitis that one can obtain.

However, you need to know that surgery is usually a final option and hardly ever needed by folks suffering from plantar fasciitis if you can take to the tips given above for your relief.

Conclusion

Thank you for downloading this book!

I hope you enjoyed reading my book? "If you enjoyed this book, don't forget to leave a review on Amazon! This way others can enjoy this book too!

I'm just a home based author with NO "big marketing company" behind me, so I highly appreciate your reviews, and it only takes a minute to do.

To submit a review:

1. Just go to Amazon and under the BOOKS category, search this book's title [Plantar Fasciitis: The Best Plantar Fasciitis Survival Guide with Special Tips on How to Manage Heel Spur and Get Plantar Fasciitis Cure Today!], to get to the product detail page for this book on Amazon.

2. Click Write a customer review in the Customer Reviews section.

3. Click Submit.

Thank you in advance for submitting. It would be greatly appreciated!"

Made in the USA
Monee, IL
23 April 2023